The Book of Supplement Secrets

A Beginner's Guide to Nutritional Supplements

Tim Mielke

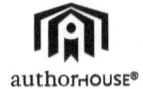

authorHOUSE®

AuthorHouse™
1663 Liberty Drive, Suite 200
Bloomington, IN 47403
www.authorhouse.com
Phone: 1-800-839-8640

First published by AuthorHouse 3/5/2009

ISBN: 978-1-4389-5615-2 (sc)

Printed in the United States of America
Bloomington, Indiana

This book is printed on acid-free paper.

Dedication

To my family and my friends who all believed in me.

Table of Contents

Introduction

Over the years, the supplement industry has been given a bad name due to unscrupulous manufacturers of inferior products, which have yielded consumers little to no results. Their primary objective was to make a quick buck off of you, the unsuspecting consumer. After you spent your hard-earned money on a nearly worthless product, they left you out to dry. If you didn't like it, it was simply too bad for you. Sure, you could always return it, but most people never even bothered. Many consumers just gave up on trying to get in shape and developed the mindset that all supplements must be worthless. Others moved on to the next nutritional craze to see where that one would take them, with the hope that it would lead to the physique of their dreams.

Through this book, my goal for you, the reader, is that you will be able to go into a health food store or on to an online supplement provider and make better purchasing decisions to get the results you want. Consider the purchase of this book an investment in your education. In the following pages, I have exposed some of the supplement industry's most devious secrets. Some you may have been able to find on your own by looking through Web sites or nutritional books. Others are hidden and not so readily available to the general public.

I have been involved in the nutrition industry for over fourteen years. In that time, I have worked for three major supplement companies. During my time with each of these companies, I was exposed to some of the dirtiest tricks that manufacturers use to make bigger profits, all while cutting back on the quality of ingredients in the products they provide. After years of advising people on which supplements to take, I realized that there were certain guidelines that I always told them to look out for. Then one day, it dawned on me that consumers could really use a book to provide guidelines that I had been explaining to clients all the while. I was not aware of any such book, so I took it upon myself to do the dirty work and go ahead and write that book! I have seen too many people get ripped off and waste their money on inferior products, myself included. I decided I wanted to use my knowledge to help you, the consumer, make better decisions on how to spend your money more effectively.

So what makes me so special that I have these insider secrets and no one else does? I am not saying that no one else does, but I have found that most of these tricks of the trade are not made readily available to the public. In fact, some are not secrets that I myself have uncovered. These are tips and tricks that I have learned from different people in the supplement industry. Some I did discover for myself, but that is not to say that no one else knew about them before I did. For example, sometimes I'd listen to someone talk about supplements; and when they said something really good that I wasn't aware of and wanted to remember, I'd write it down on a piece of paper. Eventually, I collected lots of scraps of paper with really good information. I knew something needed to be done with that information.

I'm sure some people will try to discredit me and the information in this book because I don't have any special degrees, certificates, or letters after my name. However, I do have something you can't learn in a classroom—real-world experience. I ask you—does a doctor know *everything* when you go to see him? Oftentimes you get referred to a specialist. So no, I don't know everything, nor do I claim to. But I do know these tricks of the trade, which you probably don't; otherwise, you wouldn't be reading this!

It has been said that, in order to become an expert on something, you must be consistently involved with it for at least five years. As I have said, I have been involved in this industry for over fourteen years. For eight of those years, it was my job to advise people on which supplements they should take for their own specific needs. I didn't have any certificates then, and people trusted me based on just talking to me—either on the phone or in person. I may have even talked to you, and I am asking that you trust me now.

During your reading, you will probably have questions. Maybe I can answer some of them for you now before we get too far.

I'm sure you've noticed that this book is not a gigantic encyclopedia on supplements. I could have gone on and on about the hundreds of different supplements out there, but I wanted this book to be different. I wanted this to be more of a field guide that you can use as a quick reference while you're browsing for supplements. There was no need for me to cram the pages with filler just to put out some impressively large book. In this aspect, I went for quality over quantity.

You also will notice that some of the studies conducted on the supplements were done on animals, not humans. Companies will get a lead on a possible new herb or whatnot and rush it into the lab to have tests done on rats or some other lab animal. They will see that it does show *some promise* in the animal and then quickly start an ad campaign saying they have the newest breakthrough product. Even before anything has been shown to be conclusive, they are already shoving it down our throats to buy. Mass marketing, magazine ads, posters—the whole deal. Oftentimes, it hasn't even been around long enough to see if there are any harmful side effects. I don't know about you, but I'm not a rat. Rat poison isn't tested on humans, so why do we get excited when something intended for humans proves effective in rats? Research takes time. Quality products take time to research. You cannot rush a product to the shelves and assume it will be of great quality.

You may also notice that many supplements have only one or two recent studies listed—or maybe not so recent. With so many new products coming out, it is unfeasible that a particular supplement be tested over and over. These tests all cost money! A test usually happens only when the supplement shows real promise. Otherwise, they will sit on the back burner for a while, waiting for the next promising opportunity.

It should be noted that I have not mentioned any specific product brand names or supplement companies by name. This is for legal reasons, as well as my own personal ethics. I do not want to come across as bashing any particular product or company. I simply want to expose the facts to you. It is my goal that you will be able to tell on your own who is a legitimate supplement company and whom you should stay clear of.

Also, I want you to know that it can get *expensive* to take the best supplements out there. As with anything, higher quality means higher prices. That is not to say that, just because something is the most expensive, it qualifies as the best—far from it. You could slap a price tag of $1,000 on a bucket of dirt, and it's still going to be a bucket of dirt!

Let's get one major issue out in the open. It is not—I repeat, NOT— going to be an easy ride to get you to the body of your dreams. In the age of high-speed Internet, fast food, and fast cars, we have become a society of lazy individuals. We want everything we possibly can get, and we don't want to wait for it. The supplement companies know this, and that is where they strike the hardest. They prey on our I-don't-want-to-wait attitudes and feed us misinformation to get us to buy. You *can* still get that body of your dreams, but it's going to take a lot of effort on your part. A healthy diet and an exercise program are going to serve as the foundation for it. Supplements are here to do just that—*supplement!* They are not miracle pills or powders that take all of the effort off our own backs. I know, I know, that's not a very appealing scenario, but it's a fact. Olympic athletes and the top players in your favorite sports don't get to where they are by taking the easy road.

I also want you to know that changing your body shouldn't be viewed as a diet. Diet is one of those ugly four-letter words. When people think *diet*, thoughts of eating next to nothing and starvation almost immediately pop into their heads. Along with that, there also may be many other reminders of their past failed diets and the discouragement that goes along with that failure.

Try instead to think of changing your physique as a lifestyle change. You are saying good-bye to your poor eating habits and your unhealthy body. You don't have to do this all at once like so many crash diets. I'm not asking you to give up your favorite foods but to make smarter choices when you do eat them. Instead of eating four pieces of pizza, limit yourself to two. Instead of half a bag of potato chips, eat just a handful. These are just a few tips, but the list could go on and on. Eventually, you will start to realize that you no longer crave these junk foods. Change your eating habits gradually, and you'll find that success comes much easier!

So that's enough of my soapbox speech! The time has come for us to move onto the really good stuff!

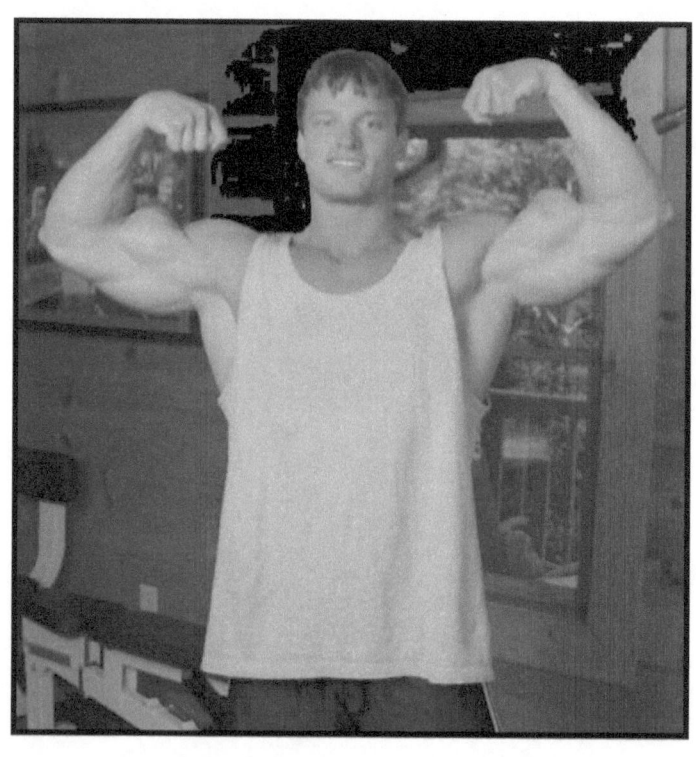

Me before my last contest.
Photo Provided By: Rick Lohre / RickLohre.com

Chapter 1: Important Terms You Should Know

I put this section first because, as you choose supplements, you will likely come across some words you are unfamiliar with. As if it weren't hard enough deciding which supplements are right for you, the terms used to explain them need an explanation themselves! I have taken the liberty of explaining these terms and phrases in a way that I hope is easy for you to understand.

Anabolic—This word is often associated with steroids (e.g., anabolic steroids), but the word simply means *pro–muscle building.* If your body is in a state of anabolism, it means you have the best internal environment for building muscle. If a product promotes anabolism, it simply means that it is designed for muscle growth.

Biological Value (BV)—This term is used to describe a food's completeness in supplying the essential amino acids and how well the food supports nitrogen retention. The standard for determining a score is egg protein, which has a score of 100. All other proteins are based on this score. The chart below outlines the BV of some of the most popular protein and carbohydrate sources.

Eggs (whole)	100
Eggs (whites)	88
Chicken, Turkey	79
Fish	70
Lean Beef	69
Milk (whole)	60
Brown Rice	57
White Rice	56
Peanuts	55
Whole Wheat	49
Whole-grain Wheat	44
Corn	36
White Potato	34

Catabolic—This term is the opposite of anabolic. This means that your body is using proteins as its primary source of fuel, which in turn results in the loss of muscle mass.

Chelated—Minerals that are chelated (key-late-ed) are bonded with another substance, usually an amino acid. Chelated minerals are more easily used by your body. A mineral must bond with an amino acid in your body in order to be absorbed properly. When minerals are chelated, your body doesn't need to supply the amino acid on its own. Chelated minerals have been said to be utilized three to five times more effectively than non-chelated ones.

Complete Protein—A protein is considered complete when it contains all of the essential amino acids. A complete protein would also have a very high biological value.

Conditionally Essential Amino Acid—An amino acid is conditionally essential when your body can manufacture it on its own; however, under periods of intense stress, the amino acid cannot be made in sufficient quantities and must be acquired through an outside source.

Cortisol—This is a very catabolic hormone your body releases during intense periods of stress.

Critical Cluster—This term is not seen too often. The critical cluster is the combination of the following five amino acids: arginine, glutamine, and the three branched chain amino acids: leucine, isoleucine, and valine. These are the most prominent amino acids used in muscle-building supplementation.

Essential Amino Acids—An essential amino acid is one that your body cannot manufacture on its own and must be obtained through an outside source (e.g., food, supplements). There are eight essential amino acids in adults and ten in children. The essential amino acids are as follows: isoleucine, leucine, valine, lysine, methionine, phenylalanine, threonine, and tryptophan. In children, arginine and histidine are essential to help support their growth.

Free Form Amino Acids—This term means that an amino acid is not bound to any other substance or another amino acid.

Glucose Level—This term refers to your amount of blood-sugar concentration. In people who are not diabetic, a normal range would run from 70 to 100 milligrams (mg) per deciliter.

Glycemic Index—This system ranks carbohydrates based on their effect on blood glucose levels. If a food is higher on the glycemic index, it will cause a larger output of insulin by the pancreas (known as a "spike"), thus rapidly increasing your blood glucose level. The scale ranges from 0 to 100, with a higher score equating to a larger output of insulin induced by the carbohydrate.

The chart below shows some healthier food choices with their ranking on the glycemic index.

Broccoli, Lettuce, Mushrooms, Onions, Red Pepper	10
Walnuts, Peanuts	15
Cherries, Cashews	22
Grapefruit	25

Kidney Beans (dried not canned)	28
Whole Milk	31
Skim Milk	32
Yams	37
Apple	38
Apple Juice, Strawberries	40
Orange, Peach	42
Sweet Potato, White Rice (long grain)	44
Grapes	46
Baked Beans	48
Oatmeal (plain), Carrots	49
Banana	52
Orange Juice, Sourdough Bread	53
Brown Rice	55
Whole Meal Rye Bread	58
Fresh Corn	60
One-minute Oatmeal	66
White Bread, White Potato (skinned)	70
Watermelon, White Rice (short grain)	72
Whole Wheat Bread	77
Rice Cakes (plain)	82
Wild Rice	87
Red Potato	88

Glycogen—Glycogen is the stored form of glucose (a sugar) in the body. It is the main short-term energy source in cells and is produced primarily in the liver and muscles. Excess glycogen that is not used for energy is stored as fat.

Insulin Resistance—This is a condition in which normal amounts of insulin are insufficient to produce a normal insulin response from fat, muscle, and liver cells. Insulin resistance results in a higher level of free fatty acids in the blood, reduces glucose uptake in muscles, and reduces glucose storage in the liver, which then results in elevated glucose levels in the blood. High levels of insulin and glucose in the blood due to insulin resistance often result in type 2 diabetes.

There are no major symptoms for insulin resistance. Blood tests are the most effective way to test for insulin resistance. Physical activities—like weight training, along with losing excess weight and healthier eating habits—are great ways to help your body better respond to insulin and reverse the negative effects of insulin resistance. Lowering your insulin resistance is a great and healthy way to help you control your weight.

Krebs Cycle—This is a complex process, so I will just explain the basic role of this cycle. *All cells* must produce energy to survive, and this is the name given to the energy production process all cells go through to produce energy. The Krebs cycle takes place within a cell's mitochondria, providing the energy needed to function and survive.

Lipotropic—Lipotropic agents are nutrients that promote the utilization of fat for energy. These nutrients can help prevent fats from accumulating in the liver, keep the arteries clear of cholesterol buildup, and help break up and redistribute fat deposits.

Nitrogen Retention—This term refers to the body's ability to hold onto nitrogen. Certain supplements can increase the body's ability to do so. Your body will either be in a positive, neutral, or negative nitrogen balance. Positive nitrogen balance means you have the proper internal environment for building muscle. A negative nitrogen balance means your body is losing muscle. A neutral balance would mean that your internal environment is not suitable for either gaining or losing muscle.

Protein Efficiency Ratio (PER)—This term is a measure of protein quality based on its ability to sustain growth in animals.

Thermogenic—This term describes those supplements used to stimulate the body's burning of fat. This is a confusing term to some, as the supplements themselves *do not* actually burn fat. These supplements work by increasing the metabolic rate, which then causes more calories to be burned. Another cause for confusion with respect to this term is that more calories burned does not necessarily equate to more fat loss. The additional calories burned could either be proteins, carbohydrates, or fats.

Chapter 2: Reading the Labels

When it comes to supplement labels, the sad truth is that many companies use a lot of fancy talk to hide the shortcomings of their products. As a consumer, the worst part about this tactic is that these companies are generally doing something *completely legal and within their rights.* Oftentimes, consumers will look at a label and think to themselves that, since the ingredient list looks to be very scientific, then the product itself must be some scientific breakthrough. More often than not, this is not the case.

Certain phrases or warnings are written on the label because the Food and Drug Administration (FDA) requires it. These warnings are discussed as well and may help you to better understand some of the FDA's regulations.

This chapter focuses on helping you understand what the label is really telling you. I 'll help you read through all the scientific terminology, so you can see what it is that you're really paying for. From there, you should be able to make smarter choices when you purchase supplements, thus saving you money and time, as well as having a much better impact on your physique.

FDA Requirements

The FDA defines supplements as "products (other than tobacco) intended to supplement the diet that bear or contain one or more of the following ingredients:

    A. a vitamin,

    B. a mineral,

    C. an herb or other botanical,

    D. an amino acid,

    E. a dietary substance for use by man to supplement the diet by increasing the total dietary intake;

    F. a concentrate, metabolite, constituent, extract, or a combination of any ingredient mentioned above."[1]

Any nutritional supplement that you buy at the store will fall into one of the above categories.

Now if a substance is found in a product only in trace amounts, then that substance's nutritional content is not required to be printed on the label. This is why you will see statements such as "May contain trace amounts of peanuts" or "This product was manufactured on equipment that processes peanuts." The peanut residue will not register enough to change the calories or the protein, carbohydrate, and fat content of the product, but it is still stated on the label due to allergen warnings. There will be more on allergens later.

The FDA requires five statements to appear on supplement labels.

---

1 Taken from the FDA's website – www.fda.gov

1. The name of the supplement.

    The product must have an identity.
2. The amount (by weight) of the supplement.

    This will be listed as the net quantity of the contents. A two-pound container should state that it weighs two pounds on the label.
3. The nutritional labeling.

    This will be listed as either Nutrition Facts or Supplement Facts.
4. The ingredient list.

    This list should state ingredients by weight from most abundant to least abundant. The individual weight of each ingredient does not need to be listed.
5. The name and place of business of the manufacturer, packer, or distributor.

Expiration Dates

Surprisingly, the FDA *does not require* expiration dates to be on any products. This may seem odd, but there is a good reason why this is not required.

The FDA's regulations are for food safety, *not food quality*. The FDA considers the *quality characteristics* of food (i.e., taste, smell, and appearance) as different from the safety characteristics (e.g., If you eat this product the way it is intended for use, will it harm you?). The quality characteristics of food largely depend on storage conditions—temperature and humidity—in the warehouse or store. If foods are kept in the best storage conditions, many foods can be considered acceptable with respect to their quality characteristics, past their expiration dates because food degradation happens very slowly.

If a tested product rolled off the manufacturing line were found to contain strychnine, this would obviously violate safety standards because it could kill you. This is an *extreme* example of food safety, but I'm just using this to get my point across about the safety characteristics of food. If it isn't safe to consume in its recommended dosage, it shouldn't even be on the shelves in the store.

If optimal storage conditions for a product have not been met—and they may differ greatly from product to product—the listed expiration date does not indicate product quality.

So, say you have a product with an expiration date set for two years from the date you purchased it. Now if you were to get it wet, let it dry out, or do anything else that it was not supposed to be exposed to or intended to have done to it, this would mean the storage conditions were compromised; it likely would be no good well before the set expiration date.

There have been some who have sent petitions to the FDA to make companies responsible for setting an expiration date, but they have been denied due to the fact that they have not shown reasonable ground to make this a regulation.

Most companies will put their own expiration date, "use by" date, lot number, or manufacturing date on their products. If it is not listed, you can always call the manufacturer to get more information on the proper storage conditions of their products or what the recommended expiration date after purchase would be.

Food Allergens

Recently, the FDA revised its labeling regulations to require any product that contains or is made from any of the eight major food allergens to declare the presence of the allergen on the label. This is confusing to many people because, for example, they will buy a product that claims to be lactose-free, yet the allergen warning says that the product contains milk.

Consider this scenario. You buy a protein powder mostly made of milk protein. We'll say that it's a whey protein powder. The label claims it is lactose-free, but the allergen warning states that it contains milk. "Wait a minute!" you say. "Milk has lactose in it!"

Before you run back to the store to exchange your product, think about this: whey protein comes from milk. (This topic is discussed in greater detail in the Protein Types section of chapter 7, but for now just take my word for it.) In order to make whey protein, you *need* milk!

So you're not buying milk, but in order to get the whey protein, it had to start as milk. I have a bottle of amino acids that I use that states on the label that the product contains milk. That's because the amino acids were derived from casein, which is part of milk protein. The same may go for any of the other food allergens.

By the way, the eight major food allergens cover the following: milk, eggs, peanuts, tree nuts (such as almonds, cashews, or walnuts), fish (such as flounder, cod, or bass), shellfish (such as crab, lobster, or shrimp), soy, and wheat.

An Important Label Statement

As you're scanning the label of your favorite protein powder, you may come across a statement that reads as follows: Use this product as a food supplement only. Do not use this product for weight reduction.

Now you ask yourself, "All those fit people in the magazines said they used this product to drop twenty pounds. Why does it say *not* to use it for weight reduction?"

Sadly, there are people out there that think that the model or spokesperson used only that product as their food source to get their incredible body. So, this person thinks to himself, "This is all I'm going to eat then."

You need to eat *real* food! A supplement cannot replace the nutritional value that you get from real foods. That is why it's called a *supplement.* It is there to *supplement* your nutritional needs, not become the entire source for them.

Serving Size

You will notice that the serving size of a protein powder may read something like *30 grams/ scoop.* As you look at the protein content per serving, you may see it only contains twenty-eight grams of protein in each scoop! What happened to the other two grams?

Slow down! They aren't trying to short you. Even though the scoop is thirty grams and the protein is twenty-eight grams (and assuming it's carb and fat free), the serving size weight still has to account for the naturally occurring trace amounts of vitamins and minerals, as well as moisture contained within the powder. So no, the manufacturers aren't trying to skimp on their end—at least not in this way. If you do come across a protein powder where the scoop weight and protein weight are exactly same, be a little wary of the manufacturer.

The Ingredient List

The first thing you need to know about the list of ingredients is that they should be listed in descending order by weight, meaning that the ingredient with the greatest amount by weight in the product should be listed first and that the rest of the ingredients should continue down the line in descending order.

So, if what you are purchasing is predominantly a protein powder, then whatever type of protein it is should be the first ingredient listed. Even if it is a blend of proteins, the most abundant protein of the blend should always come first. The blend is usually listed in parenthesis apart from the remaining ingredients.

Label Trickery

Now, here's where some companies can get really deceitful and try to trick the unsuspecting consumer into purchasing a cheaper grade of product to make a bigger profit.

I'm sure you've all read somewhere about the latest new whey protein to hit the market that will revolutionize the way you build muscle. You read the label, and it's littered with all kinds of scientific mumbo jumbo that you would need a doctorate to pronounce. To the untrained eye, these words may seem impressive, but the key is to be able to see through the hype and tell what you are really buying.

Here's an example. The label reads as follows: Cross-flow, ion-exchanged, multi-filtered premium-grade amino acid-enhanced whey protein concentrate with alpha and beta strands. (I made this up to help with my point, so don't try to find this one out there on any labels!)

Wow! That looks like something straight out of the laboratory, so it must be the good stuff. Not necessarily. Out of that entire explanation, the main thing you need to know is as follows (in bold): Cross-flow, ion-exchanged, multi-filtered premium-grade amino acid-enhanced **whey protein concentrate** with alpha and beta strands.

There are three main types of whey protein. There's concentrate, isolate, and hydrolysate. They are all explained separately in more detail under Protein Types in chapter 7 about gaining muscle. For now, here's a starter lesson.

In the example above, whey protein concentrate is the least expensive of the three types of whey protein. Generally, it is anywhere from 29 percent to 88 percent protein by weight. The rest is lactose and fat. To make a bigger profit, most companies will use the cheaper grade, meaning a lower percentage of protein, of the whey concentrate as the main source of their protein.

"But wait a minute! Wouldn't lactose then be the main ingredient?"

Unfortunately, labeling regulations do not require the contents to be labeled that way. The main ingredient is whey protein concentrate, regardless of how cheap of a grade it is. This seems wrong of the company to do this, but remember that the company has to make a profit and they are completely within their rights.

So how can you tell what concentration of whey a company is using? Unfortunately, it's not easy. Odds are that, if you start to get stomach problems from the product, it's probably cheap whey. You could always call the company and ask, but I only know of one company in the industry that doesn't use a lot of hype with its products and will give you straight answers about them.

Another trick companies use is to use a very small amount of a more expensive product—say 1 percent or 2 percent of the total weight—just to get that name on the label. This allows companies to keep their manufacturing costs down but still allows them to advertise the more expensive ingredients and charge you more for it!

Here's an example of the second instance. Say the front of the label states the product contains whey protein hydrolysate, the most expensive of the whey proteins. So you look to the ingredient list and see it is the third or fourth ingredient. (Remember, ingredients are listed by weight.) The major ingredients could be whey concentrate, then milk concentrate, and then whey hydrolysate. The hydrolysate could only be 1 percent or 2 percent of the total weight, but just to be able to advertise this costly ingredient, the company will still put it in there. This practice is completely legal, and many companies will do this not only with proteins but with many other of the more costly ingredients.

Something else that you may not be aware of is label inaccuracy. For example, a protein powder may state that there are twenty grams of protein per serving, but there really are only fifteen grams of protein per serving. You'd be upset that you were getting shorted those five grams of protein per serving. So how can you tell when this is happening?

Unfortunately, this also is not easy to figure out. You could call and ask the company if their label claims are 100 percent accurate, but the company may not give you an honest answer. Really, the only way to have this done is through expensive lab analysis. Some companies may provide you with one if you ask for it, but don't be surprised if you can't get one. The companies without anything to hide should have no problem providing this information to you.

How do companies get away with this? Unfortunately, it happens a lot more than we would like to see. The ease at which companies can hide their shortcomings makes it very difficult for us to find quality. And the amount of footwork it takes to expose these shortcomings often makes people not care. If consumers don't like the product, they jump from one to the next until they find one they like. The FDA doesn't have the manpower to police every single company to make sure they are all meeting their label claims. Once in a while, the FDA will crack down on a business, but only after a major fuss has been made about the company.

Be sure that you trust the company you prefer to buy your supplements from. Ask the representative for a copy of the label analysis. If the company is willing to provide you with one, it probably does not have anything to hide; and you are probably dealing with an honest company. If you like what you are taking and if you're getting good results, stick with what you've got.

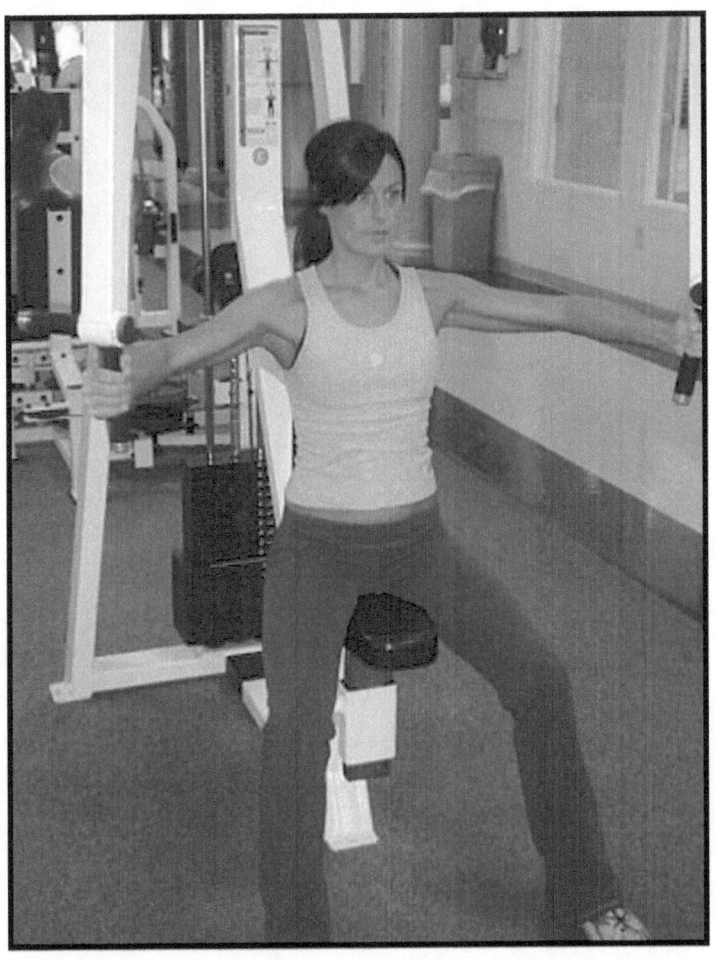

Fig. 1. Nikki Baker preps for her first contest.

Chapter 3: Marketing Tricks

The greatest products in the world will do nothing but sit on their shelves unless we know they are out there. How do they get us to notice a newcomer to the front lines of the supplement industry? Word of mouth is always a great form of advertising since you are usually getting an honest testimonial from someone you trust. On the downside, it is very slow, and supplement manufacturers don't want to wait that long for mention of their product to spread. That's where the savvy marketing gurus come in to play. They know the best and most effective ways for us to get over our fear of buying something virtually unknown and to jump onto the proverbial bandwagon.

Even those people in the marketing department have their own tricks of the trade. When you see an advertisement with before and after pictures, I want you to look carefully at the before picture. Does that person look like they work out already? Maybe they are a little out of shape, but is it relatively obvious that they have muscle underneath their flab? Are they a famous bodybuilding or fitness competitor or professional athlete? Look at the time frame of the pictures if they are provided. Generally, competitors will use twelve to sixteen weeks to get ready for a competition. Does the photo time frame fall into typical contest time? Chances are that the company took the "before" picture when they started their contest prep and then took the "after" picture the day of the show or a few days prior. The athlete was trying to get in that shape anyway!

I know of one ad that used (at the time) a famous professional fitness competitor. Her before shot was taken shortly after she just had a baby! Of course she's going to look a *little* out of shape! (Ladies, don't take this as my saying that once you're pregnant, you're automatically out of shape.) The after shot was many weeks after the birth of her baby. Her stomach had plenty of time to go back to normal, and she also had plenty of time to get her eating habits back to her old routine. Let's see—a professional fitness competitor who recently had a baby, and then weeks later she's back in shape all thanks to *one product*? This scenario just doesn't play out too well for me.

Athletes are usually paid to endorse products. There is not a lot of money in bodybuilding, even in the professional ranks. These athletes have to eat, and product endorsements help pay the bills. They are under contract to say that they take these supplements. Whether they really do is another question. A while ago, I was watching a video of a former Mr. Olympia. This video was his own production; it was not recorded for product endorsements. During a scene in his kitchen, he mixes a protein shake. In the background was a container for a supplement company well known for its quality ingredients. Was the former Mr. Olympia endorsed by them? No! He knew that company made quality products, and he had to pay for them with his own money even though he was getting paid to endorse another supplement company!

What about when we see an ad with the line "I've never felt stronger" or something along those lines? How are we as consumers supposed to react to this statement? Why would this statement make me want to buy? How am I supposed to relate to the guy in the ad? Does he feel better throughout the day or just when he gets to the gym? Is he stronger just in his bench press or all areas and lifts? Just saying "I've never felt stronger" could mean that he *feels* stronger, but it doesn't mean he *is* stronger.

Some companies have even gone so far as to using their own employees in the advertising campaign. While doing research for this book, I came across one company whose *president* was making claims that the product was great! Now, maybe it did do wonders for him, but you have to think that he has a major stake in the success of the company. Of course he's going to be biased about how well the product works. And of course, this information isn't going to be publicized in the ad. With a little diligence, however, these practices can be found out.

Also be aware of products that are promoted as either fat free or sugar free. Sometimes when a product is advertised as being fat free, it may end up being loaded with sugar! Conversely, a product that is touted as sugar free may be loaded with fat. Look at it this way—a can of Crisco is sugar free, and a bag of sugar is fat free. When a product is marketed in either of these ways, be sure to check the sugar content if it's marketed as fat free or the fat content if it's marketed as sugar free.

In reference to the calorie content of a product, many times we will come across supplements that advertise, for example, "Only three net carbs!" or some variation of that. What this means is that the company is substituting sugar alcohol for regular carbohydrates. The sugar alcohol doesn't affect your insulin levels the way normal carbs do. Thus, companies think they are getting around labeling requirements by using added sugar in their products. You may not get the insulin response from the sugar alcohol, but they still have calories and your body still has to process those calories. Just because you have a low net-carb product doesn't mean it's low-calorie. Another downside to the sugar alcohol is that in high dosages, it has been known to cause stomach and gastrointestinal (GI) distress, as well as constipation.

When flipping through the pages of your favorite health and fitness magazines, you will undoubtedly come across ads that claim that one company's product has a far greater percentage of success than the typical run-of-the-mill product. You may see statements such as, "Our new improved formula is 100 percent better than Brand X," or "I lost 33 percent more fat while using Product A." But how does one quantify these claims? How effective are they in relation to *your* goals?

Let's examine the first statement above: "Our new improved formula is 100 percent better than Brand X." Seeing that a supplement is 100 percent better than another supplement sounds impressive, right? But usually this claim is based off of one laboratory test. For instance, if the subjects were tested on their maximum repetitions on the bench press and if subject A did two repetitions while subject B did four at the same weight, then subject B did 100 percent better than subject A.

How did I come up with these numbers? Our beginning number to beat from subject A was two repetitions. If subject B also did two repetitions, he would be equal and have the same percentage or outcome as subject A. Now if subject B did three repetitions, he would have one additional rep. Since that one extra rep is half of the original two reps, subject B has done 50 percent better. Since subject B has done two extra reps, he has increased his performance by 100 percent.

This type of marketing is everywhere. When you deal with small numbers or reps as in my example, it doesn't sound all that impressive. But the supplement helped the person to get stronger. When using more complicated numbers, these types of ads are harder to figure out, and oftentimes the actual research amounts used are not listed in the ad. So how are we to know? We really can't, but it is an effective marketing ploy!

Another example from above would be the following claim: "I lost 33 percent more fat using product A." Look at this example from this perspective. If subject A lost three pounds of fat and subject B lost four pounds of fat, subject B lost the additional 33 percent—but it's only one extra pound. Now don't get me wrong; that additional pound may make all the difference in the world to subject B, but what if you needed to lose fifty pounds? That extra one pound probably will not make a huge difference.

Put yourself in the shoes of subject A in both of the above examples. Your friend and workout partner is subject B. You both take the same supplements and work out just as hard, but he's getting much more of a benefit from the supplements. He's going around the gym saying how great the supplements he's taking are. Meanwhile, you're a little angry because you aren't getting the same results. They're still working, but now it seems as though you're getting gypped. Are your supplements actually 100 percent and 33 percent worse for you?

My point is this. No one can tell you how a supplement will influence your body. You are a unique individual with your own DNA, metabolism, and hormones. I have been asked over and over, "What results will I see if I take this?" and "Will this make me look like I want to look?" Every single time I had to tell these people, "I can't answer that question." I wasn't trying to cop out of giving them an answer; I really couldn't tell them how it would work! I have no idea how that person, or any person, would react to anything. It is unreasonable to make promises to people that you cannot guarantee.

This goes along with many of the supplements I explain later in this book. Just because the research has reflected either positively or negatively about particular supplements, there is still no guarantee that they will work for you (or not work for you) in the same way. I had to go through a lot of trial and error to find out which supplements are the best for me. If you are taking a supplement and it works for you, why change it?

Chapter 4: Vitamins and Minerals

Vitamins and minerals are essential to our daily lives. They are involved in every process that goes on within our bodies. If you are just beginning a supplement regimen or simply want to take better care of yourself, vitamins and minerals should be your absolute first line of supplementation. Human beings consistently lack in any one of these nutrients, and they are all essential to our health. If you lack in any one of these micronutrients, your body is not functioning at its top level. I will not go into detail about what every single vitamin or mineral does for your body, but I will tell you some of the most important information you should know when dealing with these essential nutrients.

Keep in mind that the recommended daily allowances (RDA) are for the average person. For those of us who have stressful lives or jobs or are hard-training athletes—and really, who *doesn't* fall into one of those categories?—these daily amounts usually are inadequate to meet our demanding lifestyle. A simple *single* pill that claims to contain all of your daily vitamin and mineral needs simply will not do the job. If a pill were to contain all of your daily vitamin and mineral needs, it would be about the size of a golf ball! That's a little too hard to swallow! If you are involved in a serious weight-training schedule or you push yourself to your stress limits on a daily basis, there are plenty of vitamin and mineral packs that supply ample amounts of these nutrients for your daily needs. Just take your pack with your morning meal, and you're set for the day. It may seem like a lot of pills to swallow, but it's much easier than trying to swallow that golf ball!

For example, say you are sitting in a traffic jam, and your temper is flaring. You're rapidly burning up B and C vitamins because of your increased stress level. Or maybe you're a smoker. Your body is going to require more antioxidants to combat the effects of smoking on your body. The list can go on and on. The point is that these recommended doses really aren't enough for today's hectic lifestyle.

Some will argue that they get enough vitamins and minerals from their daily diet. First, how can you tell what amounts of vitamins and minerals you're getting from the food you eat? Very rarely is it listed, and when it is, who *really* keeps track of it all? I find it hard to believe that the people who claim they get enough from their daily diet are writing down their daily vitamin and mineral intake.

Are the foods we eat today chock-full of nutrients like they were years ago? Is the soil as rich as it used to be? Are the pesticides sprayed on the crops good for the nutritional content? There are organic foods out there; but the last time I looked, that was only a small portion of foods at the supermarket—and most people weren't buying anything from that section anyway.

The point is that, no matter how hard we try, we really can't tell the level of vitamins and minerals in our foods. We need to *supplement* to be sure we are taking in adequate nutrients. Vitamins and minerals should be the absolute *first* thing you supplement with. If we lack in one or more of these vital nutrients, our bodies are not working at their maximum efficiency; and we are not getting the maximum benefit from the remainder of our supplements. Vitamins and minerals are critical in every single function of your body.

There are two types of vitamins: water-soluble and fat-soluble.

Fat-soluble vitamins are stored in your fat cells to be used by your body when they are needed. Water-soluble vitamins are not stored within your body and can be flushed out easily. They need to be replenished on a daily basis either through food or supplements.

The B-complex vitamins would be an example of a water-soluble vitamin while vitamin A is fat-soluble.

Bioflavonoids

Often we see this word on the nutrition label of supplements accompanying vitamin C, but what are the bioflavonoids?

Bioflavonoids, also known as vitamin P, are the water-soluble plant pigments naturally found in fruits and vegetables. The term *vitamin P* has sparked some controversy because the bioflavonoids are not essential to health and are, therefore, not classified as vitamins. Your body cannot manufacture bioflavonoids, so you need to acquire them through your daily diet.

Some of the more well-known bioflavonoids include hesperin, hesperidin, eriodictyol, quercetin, and rutin. It has been reported that there are *over eight hundred different bioflavonoids!*

So what do these nutrients do? There are a wide range of advantages to supplementing with bioflavonoids. They have been shown to maintain the health of capillaries, allowing oxygen, hormones, nutrients, and antibodies to pass from the bloodstream into individual cells. If your capillaries are too fragile, blood may drain into the individual cell. A sign of capillary weakness would be easy bruising.

Bioflavonoids also have been shown to aid in blood-clotting disorders, combating free radicals; they are also anti-inflammatory, antihistaminic, and antiviral.

Bioflavonoids are often found in supplements in conjunction with vitamin C because they help to protect vitamin C, enhance its longevity, and increase its absorption. They are also found in many of the same foods as vitamin C. Some foods high in bioflavonoids are apricots, blackberries, broccoli, cantaloupe, cherries, grapefruits, grapes, oranges, and lemons.

Although there is no recommended daily dosage of the bioflavonoids, 500 mg per day of any combination of them is the usual recommendation. The only negative side effect I've come across is that very high doses of bioflavonoids have been known to cause diarrhea. Other than that, they appear to be perfectly safe.

Chapter 5: Essential Fatty Acids

More commonly referred to as EFAs, essential fatty acids are Omega-3, Omega-6, and Omega-9. Omega-3 is often supplemented in the form of linolenic acid, Omega-6 as linoleic acid, and Omega-9 as oleic acid—although there are other forms. These fatty acids are referred to as essential because your body cannot manufacture them on its own, and they must be obtained through your daily diet or nutritional supplementation. (Note: Omega-9 is a necessary fatty acid, but it is technically not essential. This is because our bodies can manufacture modest amounts of this fat on their own as long as there are sufficient amounts of the other two EFAs present.)

EFAs have a wide array of functions they are involved with in the human body, and a deficiency in any one of them can lead to myriad negative side effects. EFAs are involved in many functions of the cardiovascular, reproductive, immune, and nervous systems. We need EFAs to make and repair cell membranes; provide adequate nutrition to cells; expel harmful waste products; regulate heart rate, blood pressure, and blood clotting; aid in immune function by helping our bodies fight infection, among other critical functions. EFAs have functions in nearly all tissues.

So how do the EFAs aid you in your quest for the perfect body? The EFAs will help aid your metabolism by increasing fat usage for energy, as well as preventing ingested fats from being turned into stored body fat.

Let's get a little more in-depth with each of the EFA's specific effects on your metabolism.

Omega-3

Omega-3s have been shown to increase insulin sensitivity substantially. Increased sensitivity to insulin means that your body will have a much greater anabolic response to insulin, increasing your ability to burn fat while keeping your body in a much better internal anabolic environment. As we've read previously, an internal anabolic environment is what we want when we are trying to gain more muscle.

In one study with diabetic subjects, it was shown that, with just three grams of Omega-3s per day over eight weeks, the subjects had increased insulin sensitivity and lower plasma triglyceride levels. This means that their bodies were producing insulin more efficiently, and there was fewer fatty acids circulating through the bloodstream.

Omega-3s also have shown that they greatly increase thermogenesis, which in turn burns more calories and can aid in the reduction of body fat.

An additional benefit of Omega-3s is that they aid in repairing joint damage and reduce inflammation. For this reason, you may see Omega-3s in the ingredient list of some joint care supplements. I don't know anyone who lifts weights and who doesn't have some sort of joint discomfort, myself included!

Omega-6

Omega-6s also aid in lowering cholesterol levels. Like the Omega-3s, they also increase thermogenesis and the use of fat as energy. They play a large role in the maintenance of the cardiovascular system as well.

It should be noted that Omega-6s, in high dosages, have shown an *adverse effect* on insulin sensitivity and may, in fact, lead to insulin resistance and its many serious side effects. One study showed that the subjects who were given diets high in Omega-6s actually developed insulin resistance. However, a small percentage—11 percent of total fatty intake—of Omega-3s were then substituted into the regimen. The result was that the addition of the Omega-3s normalized the response of insulin in the subjects. It would seem that, if you supplement with Omega-6s, you want to be sure to include Omega-3s to keep them in check—as the two work better together than separately.

Omega-9

Since Omega-9s can be manufactured by your body, I won't go into great detail about this one. If you supplement the other two EFAs, it may not be necessary to supplement with Omega-9s although this EFA is often found alongside the others on many nutrition labels.

Omega-9s aid your cardiovascular system by lowering your risk of heart attack. Also, they reduce the risk of arteriosclerosis, or the hardening of the arteries. Preventing arteriosclerosis allows for easier passage of blood through the arteries. Omega-9s also have been shown to aid in cancer prevention.

Supplementing with EFAs

It should be noted that there are certain guidelines that should be followed when taking supplemental EFAs.

First, high heats can destroy EFAs. High heats can even change the *chemical structure* of the EFAs, which makes them useless. If you cook using an oil rich in EFAs, it is best to use one that can withstand the heat without destroying the sensitive EFAs within. Extra virgin olive oil, which I use, and grapeseed oil can tolerate high heats very well. Another option would be to add the oil after you have cooked your food.

Exposure to air can also cause rapid deterioration of EFAs. Of course it would be impossible to get the oil out of the container and into your stomach without air reaching it, but just be sure you close the lid tight; and don't leave it open for too long.

Light exposure also will have a negative effect on the oil. Keep them in a dark cupboard or use an opaque container.

There are many sources of EFAs. They may be purchased in capsules from your local nutrition store, but here are a few whole food sources where you can find naturally occurring EFAs.

Omega-3—Flax (oil, seeds, and meal), walnuts, pumpkin seeds, Brazil nuts, sesame seeds, avocados, canola oil, soybean oil, salmon, mackerel, sardines, and albacore tuna. Flaxseed oil has the highest amount of linolenic acid in any food.

Omega-6—Flax (oil, seeds, and meal), grapeseed oil, pumpkin seeds, pistachios, olive oil, olives, raw sunflower seeds, borage oil, evening primrose oil, and black currant seed oil.

Omega-9—Olive oil (extra virgin or virgin), olives, avocados, almonds, peanuts, sesame oil, pecans, pistachios, cashews, and macadamia nuts.

There are more sources than just these listed here. Check out a nutritional book specific to the EFAs for more sources.

A *minimum* daily intake ratio of Omega-6 and Omega-3 should be about 1.5 grams of each. Keeping these EFAs at a ratio of 1:1 would be ideal and should be sufficient so as not to cause any negative side effects from an overabundance of Omega-6s. Also, this level of supplementation would provide sufficient EFAs to make additional Omega-9 supplementation unnecessary.

Medium Chain Triglycerides

In addition to the essential fatty acids, medium chain triglycerides (MCT) are also a class of fatty acids, which are used as an additional source of energy. MCTs are given the name of medium chain because their chemical structure is shorter in length than most other fats and oils. MCTs also have a slightly lower calorie content of 8.3 calories per gram compared to longer chain fatty acids of nine calories per gram.

MCTs have a better absorption rate than other fatty acids and show some resemblance to carbohydrates in that they are burned more quickly for energy. This quick absorption rate provides a boost of energy to a person and helps increase the metabolic rate. Since these fatty acids are used as an energy source, they spare your glycogen from being used initially. Sparing glycogen may increase endurance and improve performance.

Usually these fats are used by endurance athletes for a sustained form of energy. In a study conducted on cyclists, each rider was either given an MCT solution, a typical carbohydrate sports drink, or a mixture of MCTs and the sports drink. They were first told to cycle at 70 percent of their maximum for two hours. After that initial ride, they immediately rode an additional forty-kilometer time trial for about another hour. Those who drank the combination of MCTs and the sports drink cycled the fastest and the farthest.

A friend of mine, who is an endurance athlete involved in cage fighting, told me that when he prepares for his fights, he sometimes uses MCTs and notices a significant improvement in his endurance. I've seen his training folks. It will boggle your mind at how these guys push themselves to their physical limit day after day. If someone training this intensely notices a significant difference while using a supplement, it must be doing its job!

Since MCTs can aid in a metabolic increase, it was thought that they would also aid in weight loss. Research on this is limited, however, it is *estimated* that the amount of calories needed from MCTs to have any significant effect on weight loss would be almost 50 percent of a person's total caloric intake.

A study related to MCTs and weight loss was conducted with obese women and a calorie-restricted diet. Of their total caloric intake, roughly 24 percent was from MCTs. After three months of that high percentage, subjects experienced no greater fat loss than when regular fats were used.[2]

To have the desired benefit, MCTs are best used on a daily basis instead of as a onetime shot before a meet or a competition. Athletes probably will not benefit from less than fifty grams per day, but such large doses may lead to gastrointestinal (GI) problems. This situation can be avoided by taking MCTs with carbohydrates or by dividing the doses throughout the day.

MCTs can be found in coconut oil, palm kernel oil, butter, and, by themselves as a liquid supplement.

---

[2] American Journal of Clinical Nutrition - 1989

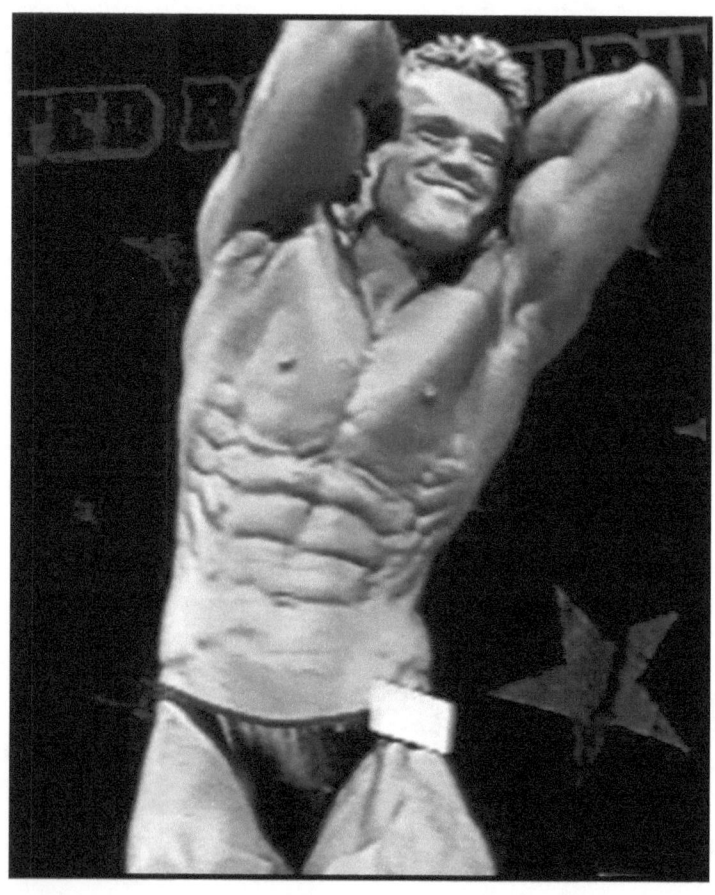

Fig. 2. Sean Young has mastered the art of fat loss.

Chapter 6: Fat Loss

Fat loss could possibly be the most confusing and frustrating area for just about anyone who wants to improve his or her physique. There are so many outrageous claims that the latest fat-loss miracle will turn your body around overnight that it makes it very difficult to believe any of them. There are some staple supplements that have been tried and true and really do work well. Others get sold in the marketplace without proper testing to see if they really are effective. Here are a few things you need to know about fat-loss supplements.

First and most importantly, these products are *always* to be used in conjunction with proper diet and exercise. I know, I know. It's not very appealing that we actually have to put forth some effort on our part to accomplish our goals. But it doesn't matter how great a product is, you cannot realistically expect to eat whatever you want whenever you want and still maintain a great-looking body. Think about it—you might not be a competitive bodybuilder or even want to be, but those people do not look the way they do from supplements alone. Steroids? I cannot deny that they are part of the bodybuilding culture, but I have known plenty of lifetime natural competitors who have amazing physiques without steroids. The key is that they know what supplements to take to help fuel their diet and efforts in the gym. The old saying, "You are what you eat" has never been more true.

Think about this scenario. Let's say you've recently purchased a high-performance sports car. The owner's manual calls for a high-octane premium gas. Sooner or later, you decide that you want to save a few bucks on gas, and you put the cheaper fuel in your sports car. You'll soon notice that your engine idles strangely and that you don't accelerate quite as quickly as you used to. Your expensive high-performance sports car isn't performing as highly as it should be. What happened? It's quite simple. You tried to skimp on the gas, and your engine paid the price! It was designed to use the higher-octane gas.

The human body functions in quite the same manner as that high-performance sports car. When you eat junk food, your body doesn't perform as optimally as it should. You feel tired and sluggish throughout the day. You can't think as clearly. You get sugar cravings and hunger pangs. Instead of putting the higher-quality, more nutritious food in your body and working out, you opted for the junk food while watching TV on the couch—and look what has happened. Your physique ended up paying the price!

The second thing you should know is that there are certain dosages used in research to test the effectiveness of a product. You need to be sure you are taking the proper amount to get the most out of your supplements. If the research on a particular product shows a dosage of 1,000 mg, and you buy a product that contains only

100 mg, chances are you are not going to get much of an effect. Here's the kicker, though—many companies will still advertise that the product contains the popular ingredient. (Remember the label tricks from earlier in chapter 2?) In general, people don't know what amounts the research supports for the supplement to be effective. So they buy it; it doesn't work and they get upset. When this starts to happen over and over again, no wonder people think that the supplement industry is a joke.

Let's talk about another common cause of confusion when it comes to fat loss. Oftentimes people confuse *weight loss* with *fat loss*. In many advertisements, people boast of losing up to thirty pounds in one week! While this is extremely hard to do—and not to mention dangerous—losing thirty pounds that rapidly is *not* going to be entirely fat loss. The majority of this weight loss is going to come from water. While we do want to lose *excess* water, this is not going to be the key to attain the body of your dreams. With fat loss, excess water loss comes along with it. Muscle loss will also occur in such dramatic weight changes. If you want to maximize your fat loss while retaining lean muscle, a slower and more gradual decline is the preferred and healthier, method. A rule of thumb is one to two pounds of fat loss per week. You may experience slightly more or less than these amounts based on your own personal genetics, as well as how vigorously you adhere to a proper diet and exercise routine.

The Most Popular of the Fat-Loss Supplements

Some of the supplements listed below have been proven to be effective in aiding fat loss *along with proper diet and exercise*. Others are rapidly gaining popularity, but the final say on whether they have been proven effective is still out.

7-keto DHEA

The supplement 7-keto DHEA is a metabolite (a conversion product) of DHEA. Once DHEA is converted into 7-keto DHEA in your body, it works together with your thyroid and thermogenic liver enzymes to increase your calorie-burning rate. This means that your natural metabolism gets a little kick-start. Burning more calories means more fat loss! The great thing about 7-keto DHEA is that it helps your body burn more calories while at rest. So even while you're just sitting at work or in the car, your metabolism is burning more calories than it used to. Imagine how many more calories you'll be burning up while you're pumping iron or running on the treadmill! With 7-keto DHEA your body is transformed into a calorie-burning furnace!

Supplemental 7-keto DHEA is nonhormonal and has been proven safe and effective in many clinical studies. The effective clinical dosage used in testing 7-keto DHEA is 200 mg per day.

Carnitine

Carnitine is a *conditionally essential* amino acid. The main function of carnitine is metabolizing fat. Carnitine metabolizes fat by utilizing fatty acids as a source of energy for muscle cells.

Muscles burn both fat and glycogen for energy. When you supplement with sufficient amounts of carnitine, your body shifts to primarily using fat as its source for energy production. This change allows both your muscles and your liver to retain their glycogen stores, giving them more endurance for those intense workouts.

Carnitine also has been shown to enhance your muscles' ability to maintain the uptake of branched chain amino acids (BCAA). This means more strength, longer muscular endurance, and an increased look of hardness to your muscles when they are supplemented together.

Don't be fooled by labels that claim to have carnitine as an ingredient. Oftentimes, the amount is so small it does you no good. The minimum dose for carnitine to be effective is 1,000 mg–1,200 mg daily.

Carnitine supplements cannot be exposed to moisture. This causes a rapid deterioration of the amino acid, rendering it ineffective. Avoid liquid products that boast carnitine as a primary ingredient. Don't believe me? Try setting a tablet of carnitine out on the table overnight. By morning, the moisture in the air will have started to break down the tablet. It will start to look cracked and brittle. If that's just from one night of exposure, imagine what happens when carnitine is sitting in water for days or weeks!

Carnitine is absolutely one of my favorite supplements for fat loss. It helps to get me in my best shape without any jitters or other side effects. I love to combine it with 7-keto DHEA. That way, I know I'm hitting fat loss with a double attack!

Chromium Picolinate

This is a combination of the mineral chromium and picolinic acid. Chromium can be difficult for your body to absorb in sufficient quantities by itself, so it is often chelated with picolinic acid to make it more readily absorbed and usable by your body.

Chromium helps the absorption of nutrients through insulin regulation. Keeping insulin levels stable is a key factor in weight management. Stable insulin levels also help keep energy levels consistent, as well as your appetite and mood. Additionally, chromium can help in the prevention and lowering of high blood pressure.

While there is no recommended dosage of Chromium Picolinate, the general amount used is 200 mcg.

Hydroxycitric Acid

Another wildly popular supplement to come onto the weight-loss scene is hydroxycitric acid, also known as HCA. HCA is the active ingredient in the plant *Garcinia cambogia*. In Indian and Thai food, it is used as a flavoring agent and as a condiment. In Indian folk medicine, a tea or dried powder form is used as a laxative and to aid in combating rheumatism.

To help those of us who want to get rid of excess body fat, HCA is believed to inhibit the body's ability to store fat that is ingested. This means that more of the fats from your foods are excreted rather than stored as body fat. It is also believed to aid the body in its use of stored body fat as its energy source. It may also help reduce appetite.

In studies conducted on rats, HCA supplementation has been shown to reduce their overall food intake. The lowering of the caloric intake led to subsequent weight loss. Studies also showed that it also slowed the digestion of sugars. Sugars normally digested in about twenty minutes were slowed to over two hours after HCA supplementation. A slower digestion of sugar means a more stable output of insulin, which, in turn, helps keep sugar cravings in check, as well as a more stable level of energy throughout the day.

A study conducted with human subjects involved 135 volunteers. Subjects received either 1,500 mg of HCA or a placebo and had their dietary intake restricted. After twelve weeks, subjects in *both* groups lost a significant amount of weight. The result of this study was that HCA failed to do anything more than aid in weight loss.

The range of dosages of HCA used in human studies is anywhere from 250 mg to 1,000 mg three times per day. HCA has not been shown to have any negative side effects.

While the studies on animals look very promising, there simply isn't enough evidence to prove that HCA would be effective in humans. There are studies that support that HCA is effective in aiding humans, but the evidence has not recurred regularly enough to prove it conclusive.[3] With its ability to slow sugar digestion, HCA would seem a likely candidate to pair with Chromium Picolinate.

Hoodia
Quite possibly the most talked about weight-loss supplement in recent years, hoodia has exploded onto the weight-loss scene with some great possibilities.

---

[3] International Journal of Obesity (1999); Open Field, Physician Controlled, Clinical Evaluation of Botanical Weight Loss Formula (1995)

For hundreds of years, the San Bushmen of the Kalahari Desert in South Africa have been using hoodia as an appetite suppressant when they would go on long hunting trips, in which both water and food would be scarce. Aside from its appetite-suppressing abilities, the Bushmen also said eating hoodia would help increase their energy levels. Another great benefit when you're out on a long hunting trip!

The first research of hoodia didn't take place until the 1960s. After another thirty years, South African labs were finally able to isolate the specific appetite-suppressing agent. This agent has been given the name of P57. Only from the P57 molecule can you get the appetite-suppressing effects of hoodia.

The P57 molecule works by imitating the way glucose affects your brain. Your brain will be fooled into thinking that you are full when your stomach is not. (Don't take this as a way to completely starve yourself from all food. Not only is it completely unhealthy to starve yourself, but your body will figure it out sooner or later that it isn't full.) The basis behind hoodia is that you can curb *cravings* for snacks and junk food.

The research is sparse, but it all looks to be very positive on hoodia. In one study, overweight volunteers were given P57 or a placebo and told to continue their normal diet. Those taking P57 showed significant fat loss and an overall reduction in caloric intake (on average eating 1,000 calories less *per day*!) and no side effects.[4] Another study over fifteen days with nine volunteers involved either a placebo or P57. Those using P57

---

[4] Study conducted by Phytopharm (2001)

experienced greater fat loss. Animal studies also showed that hoodia had a positive effect on weight loss due to lower calorie consumption.[5]

Unfortunately, the process involved to harvest hoodia is very expensive. One major pharmaceutical company wanted to make a synthetic version of P57 as a way to make a less expensive supplement from the hoodia plant. This turned out to be a wasted effort as the process turned out to be very costly as well.

There are certain things you should look or ask for when you purchase your hoodia supplement to ensure you are getting a legitimate product.

First, your hoodia should come from the *Hoodia gordonii* plant. There are more than twenty different species of hoodia plants, but only the *Hoodia gordonii* species has been shown to have appetite-suppressing effects. This is something you want to watch out for if the company is advertising 100 percent hoodia. Just by stating "100 percent hoodia" on the labels is not enough. It needs to say "100 percent *Hoodia gordonii*".

Second, do not buy anything that uses hoodia that was not grown in the Kalahari Desert. Hoodia needs a very hot climate to mature, and even then it can take four to five years. Others have tried to grow the plant in the United States and other countries, but it simply doesn't work because the climate isn't right. Another trick is to use *Hoodia gordonii* seeds from the Kalahari (and state this on the label), but then grow the seeds in another country. Again, this process will not get the desired results

---

[5] Council for Scientific and Industrial Research (1996)

with the hoodia because the seeds were not grown in the proper climate.

Next, be on the lookout for label claims that state they use the whole hoodia plant. The P57 molecule is only found in the *heart* of the plant. If you're using the whole plant to make a pill from, there's a lot of additional waste that just takes up space.

Also, any company that legally harvests hoodia from the San Bushmen has to pay them royalties. Hoodia is a protected plant, and the farms that grow it are controlled by the government. You need a permit to export the plant since it is protected by the government. The Convention on the International Trade in Endangered Species of Wild Fauna and Flora (CITES) issues permits to those who are allowed to export hoodia. Check with your supplement company to ensure they have these documents or are buying their hoodia from an approved company.

A certain pharmaceutical giant—we'll call them Company X—has a patent on the use of *Hoodia gordonii* as a weight-loss supplement and the process to extract the plants, so anyone that wants to use it in their products must get their approval first. If a provider of hoodia bypasses this step, they're not obtaining hoodia legally.

So how are all these other companies getting away with putting hoodia on their bottles? It is a complicated legal matter. Basically, companies can sell *Hoodia gordonii* as a supplement, but they *cannot* state that it can be used for weight loss or as an appetite suppressant.

As you can see, all these factors involved can cause a lot of trouble for supplement manufacturers that just want to sell hoodia and make money. The harvesting process, the royalties, and permission costs can add up. If a company is selling hoodia cheaply, odds are you don't have a legitimate hoodia product. This may be a lot of hassle to go through when you look for hoodia, but isn't it better than getting ripped off completely?

The downside of hoodia is that no one has found a set dosage to be effective. Your dosage will be based on your own personal genetics; it will be different for everyone else. You will need to experiment on your own to find out which dosage works the best for you. As of yet, no negative side effects about hoodia have been reported.

Alpha-Lipoic Acid

Alpha-Lipoic Acid, or ALA as it is commonly called, is a fatty acid found naturally inside every cell in the human body. ALA plays a vital role in the Krebs cycle of energy production in cells. ALA works by converting glucose into energy. Our bodies actually make enough ALA on their own to provide for this function.

In the 1980s, ALA was discovered to also be a powerful antioxidant. The drawback to this effect, though, is that ALA only serves as an antioxidant when there is an abundance of it circulating freely in the bloodstream. Unfortunately, unless we are using supplemental ALA, there is a minimal amount that naturally circulates in the bloodstream.

On the positive side, ALA's uniqueness is that its antioxidant properties function in both the fatty and watery regions of cells and has been shown to combat a significant number of free radicals.[6] This is a huge

---

[6] Free Radical Biology and Medicine (1995)

advantage over such popular antioxidants as vitamin E and vitamin C. What I mean by this is that the water-soluble vitamin C will attack free radicals in the watery regions of cells while the fat-soluble vitamin E will attack only those free radicals in the fatty regions. Besides attacking free radicals in both areas, ALA also extends the lifespan of vitamins C and E.

ALA has also been shown to aid those in their quest for fat loss. It may improve blood-sugar regulation and has been shown to reduce insulin resistance. ALA has been shown to speed the removal of glucose from the bloodstream through its ability to enhance insulin function. Keeping your insulin levels stable is very important in fighting sugar cravings, as well as the energy swings that may accompany them.

Aside from the normal supplemental forms of ALA, it is also found in very small amounts in foods such as spinach, broccoli, peas, and brussels sprouts.

Although research and evidence have grown to suggest the importance and the benefits of ALA, there is no recommended dosage. In one study, subjects were given 600 mg, 1,200 mg, or 1,800 mg per day of ALA. After five weeks, all doses of ALA reversed the test subjects' symptoms. However, the 600 mg per day was tolerated the best. Again, you will need to figure out the dosage right for you.

Some noted side effects in the higher range of doses are headache, a tingling sensation, skin rash, or muscle cramps.

Conjugated Linoleic Acid (CLA)

Conjugated linoleic acid (CLA) is a healthy fat with many promising benefits. Our bodies cannot produce CLA, so we must obtain it through outside sources. Other than supplements, some sources with the highest concentration of CLA include whole milk, butter, and beef; but unfortunately, these are also high sources of fat.

CLA has been touted as a fat reducer and muscle-building aid. However, one study has shown that it doesn't actually help make fat cells smaller (body fat reduction); it simply prevents them from getting bigger. The obese subjects used in this study were put on a controlled diet and supplemented with approximately 3.5 grams of CLA per day. After they ended their dieting phase, the subjects gained back any weight they had lost while supplementing with CLA. On the positive side, those who did supplement with CLA had a higher chance of gaining muscle instead of fat.[7]

Additional benefits to CLA supplementation include an improved metabolic rate, a decrease in abdominal fat, enhanced muscle growth, lower cholesterol and triglycerides, lower insulin resistance, and an improved immune system function.

What many people don't know is that there are sixteen different types of CLA. According to research, each has its own benefits. What each individual one does is beyond the scope of this book.

One major drawback of CLA is the synthetic version advertised as the weight-loss aid and muscle builder. Research on this synthetic version has shown that it

[7] University of Wisconsin-Madison (2000)

can actually do more harm than good. Some of the negative side effects include promoting insulin resistance, elevating glucose levels, and decreasing HDL, the good cholesterol.[8]

If you supplement with CLA, research points to the natural form as your best bet. The meat and dairy products of grass-fed, not grain-fed, animals has been shown to be the most abundant source of natural CLA. If you are going to use the pill form of CLA, it's probably best if you make sure it is in its natural version, not the synthetic one. The form should be stated on the label, or you can ask the manufacturer.

The final ruling on CLA is still out, but the natural version is showing serious promise. There is no daily recommended dose of CLA, but research would suggest about three to four grams per day.

Chitosan
Chitosan comes from chitin, a polysaccharide (complex carbohydrate) found in shellfish.

The world's quest for a miracle weight-loss pill was thought to have come to an end when chitosan first came on the scene. This supplement boasted claims of "Eat whatever you want and still look great!" and "Never exercise again!" Chitosan was rushed to the market with the premise that it would block your body from absorbing the fat in your diet, which would cause it to be excreted. Though chitosan can decrease the amount of fat absorption, there is no evidence that it is effective for weight loss.

---

[8] Journal of Lipid Research (2003)

One study on chitosan has found that the amount of fat actually blocked from absorption is too small to make a difference. This study used fifteen men who consumed five meals with a total of twenty-five grams of fat per day. It was found that, while taking chitosan for four days, the amount of fat excreted was increased by about one gram! That's only a nine calorie difference per day! Granted, these subjects were only eating twenty-five grams of fat per day, but one gram represents only 4 percent of the total fat intake in the study. Adjust that on a larger scale, and that's only four grams out of one hundred, equating to only thirty-six calories blocked from absorption.

Another study took thirty overweight subjects and gave them either chitosan or a placebo for twenty-eight consecutive days. During this time they were told to eat their normal diet. After that time, the group taking the chitosan showed no differences in either weight or serum cholesterol levels compared to the group taking the placebo.

A few years back, the FDA had to tell one company to stop making claims that its products containing chitosan would reduce the risk of obesity, high blood pressure, heart attack, and cancer. On top of that, the Federal Trade Commission (FTC) won an $8.3 million settlement against another highly publicized company because of its false claims about its products with chitosan. These companies were actually claiming that their chitosan *would* improve health in the ways described above. In the supplement industry, it's a no-no to make claims that any product will get you results. All the companies can do is state that they *may* help you accomplish your goals.

On top of all this, another drawback is that chitosan comes from shellfish, which is one of the eight major allergens. So if you fall into the category of those allergic to shellfish, chitosan would not work for you.

There is very little evidence that suggests chitosan is an effective fat-loss supplement. Until that time comes, your best bet is to put your money into other proven weight-loss supplements.

Growth Hormone Stimulators

Growth hormone (GH) is a hormone secreted by the pituitary gland that aids in muscle gain and fat loss by aiding muscles' uptake of protein for lean mass gains and by breaking down fats for energy. GH is abundant in children and teens, but production drops significantly as we age (although it is still stored in the pituitary gland).

The purpose of these GH stimulators is to get the pituitary gland to release its stores of GH, so there is more of the hormone circulating throughout your bloodstream. This is especially important as we get older. The more GH that is active in your bloodstream, the easier it is for you to gain muscle and lose fat. GH is a potent fat-loss agent and has been reported to have anti-aging effects.

There are two predominant amino acid combinations that are the most effective for stimulating a GH release. They are arginine with lysine and arginine with ornithine; arginine being the most important of the three.

Arginine

Arginine is a conditionally essential amino acid. It is mainly produced in the kidneys. Arginine is used in several functions of the body, including removal of ammonia from the body and the formation of compounds like nitric oxide (NO) and creatine. NO reduces stiffness in the blood vessels, helps to increase blood flow, and improves blood vessel function. (The function of NO is better explained in chapter 7.)

Arginine has a variety of uses other than stimulating GH output. It can aid in treating heart disease and erectile dysfunction and may also speed up the process of wound healing.

A typical dosage of arginine for GH release is 2000 mg–3000 mg per day. It is best taken on an empty stomach. However, this may cause stomach discomfort because arginine can also increase the production of stomach acid.

Ornithine aids in the metabolism of arginine and is usually taken in a similar dosage. Alone, this amino acid will not do much for GH production.

Lysine also greatly increases the ability of arginine to produce GH. One study showed that the combination of these two amino acids *in equal doses* was ten times more effective than taking arginine alone.

Citrulline

Citrulline is also a non-essential amino acid, which means that your body can manufacture enough on its own. Citrulline works by increasing the rate at which toxic byproducts of exercise (i.e., lactic acid and ammonia) are removed from the muscle. Removing these waste materials from your body more quickly and more efficiently means that you will be able to train longer and harder, as well as improve your recovery time.

Another huge benefit of citrulline supplementation is that it extends the life of arginine. . This is important because as you read previously, it plays a major role in the production of nitric oxide. When you add citrulline to the formula, you get an extended life to your "pump" and vascularity! Since it helps with the production of nitric oxide, citrulline may also increase cardiovascular health, as well as aid in sexual function by the increased blood flow.

The dosage range of citrulline is anywhere from two to six grams per day. If you are using it in conjunction with arginine, the optimal time is thirty to forty minutes before exercise.

Gamma-aminobutyric Acid

More commonly referred to as GABA, Gamma-aminobutyric Acid is the most important inhibitory neurotransmitter (i.e., chemical messenger) in the brain. GABA is made *in the brain* by the amino acid glutamic acid along with vitamin B6. GABA is actually an amino acid, but it is classified as a neurotransmitter. GABA helps induce relaxation, analgesia, and sleep. When the brain gets too excited, GABA is able to calm it down.

GABA works by stimulating the pituitary gland into producing more growth hormone. Again, higher growth hormone output aids in combating aging, helps reduce body fat, and aids in increasing muscle.

GABA supplements have somewhat gone by the wayside, but studies have shown that it effectively increases growth hormone levels significantly. A study done on thirty-seven subjects, nineteen of whom were given five grams of GABA versus eighteen subjects who were given a placebo, shows that, after ninety minutes, the growth hormone levels in those given GABA had *increased by 500 percent!*

Dosages range between two grams and eighteen grams; taking more than eighteen grams tends not to provide any additional benefit and can be very expensive.

Some side effects from taking GABA include a mild tingling sensation and a brief change in heart rate or breathing patterns, which should quickly disappear and have been shown not to be harmful. Since GABA helps induce relaxation and sleep, the optimal time to take it would be about thirty to sixty minutes before going to bed.

Other Supplements to Aid Fat Loss

Methionine
Methionine is an essential amino acid. This is one of the lipotropics, along with choline and inositol, which aid the liver in the production of lecithin. Lecithin prevents fat from accumulating in the liver, helps keep the arteries clear of cholesterol deposits, and aids in the breakdown and redistribution of fatty acids. Supplemental lecithin is also available at your local nutrition store.

Choline
Choline is considered part of the family of B-complex vitamins, but it is not a B vitamin itself. It is also a

---

[9] First Medical Clinic – University of Milan

lipotropic and aids in the metabolism of fats, helps keep arteries clean, and helps reduce cholesterol buildup. Often you will find choline paired with inositol.

Inositol
This is also considered part of the B-complex vitamins, but it is not considered a B vitamin itself. It is also a lipotropic, and aids in the metabolism of fats and cholesterol and in cholesterol reduction.

* * *

So there you have a few of the most popular and some of the most effective supplements to help fight fat. Using combinations of the most proven supplements is usually more effective that just using one supplement alone. That way, you are attacking unsightly fat from multiple angles, greatly increasing your chances of success, and getting the body you have always wanted. Plus, you won't be wasting your time and hard-earned money on ineffective junk!

Again, these products should be used in conjunction with good eating habits and an exercise routine. I cannot stress that enough. Supplements alone will not get you where you want to be!

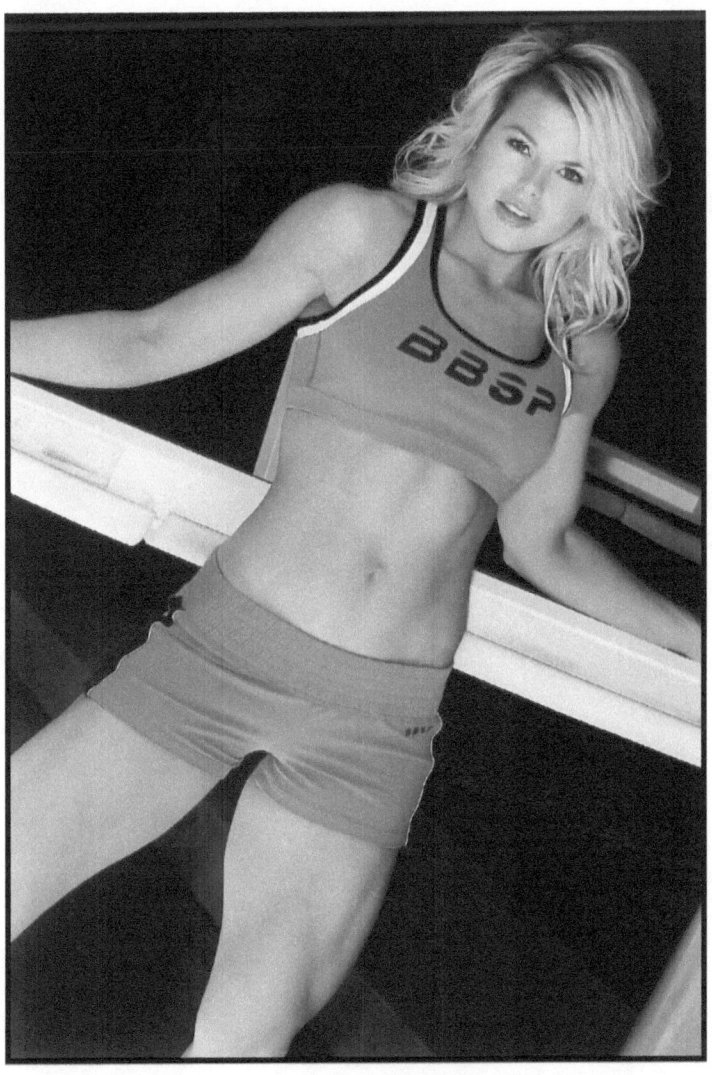

*Fig. 3. Stephanie Billings combines
both muscularity and femininity.
Photo courtesy of Kelly Beach.
www.kellybeachphoto.com*

Chapter 7: Gaining Muscle

Before we go any further in this chapter, I want to take a minute to talk to all of the ladies out there. Throughout my years in this industry, one recurrent theme that seems to scare most women with whom I have spoken is the fear of getting bulky. They think that if they start to lift weights, then they are automatically going to pack on pounds of muscle virtually overnight and start to resemble a man. Time and again, my answer to these women was always, "You are not a man."

Ladies, you do not have the internal hormonal environment to gain the amount of muscle that men can. While you *do* have testosterone, the dominant male hormone, circulating in your body, the average amount in women is a small fraction of what men have. Thus, we have an easier time adding muscle in general. There are some women who have a naturally higher testosterone level than other women, but again it is not as significant as a man's level.

I also have spoken with some women who have told me they are scared to lift weights because they claim they add muscle "way too easy." My advice to them (and you) is the following: when you get to a point where you like the way your body looks, stop adding weight to the amounts you lift. Staying at a steady lifting weight will cause your muscles to stabilize their growth. Muscles grow when they are forced to compensate for added weight.

It is possible to be *feminine* and *muscular* at the same time. Just take a look at the pictures of the women in physique magazines. They combine both beauty and muscularity. However, there are exceptions to this as well. Don't let the pictures of *overly muscular* women scare you. Odds are that they are *not natural!*

So think about this the next time you debate whether or not you want to go lift weights. What shapes the curves of a woman's body? Muscle! Fat just hangs there! If you want a perfect figure, you need to train those muscles to hold that shape!

And guys, *some* of the above can go for you as well. If you like the amount of muscle you have, don't increase your lifting weight. If you want a "manly" physique, train your muscles to hold that shape. Also, don't think that just because you've started to lift weights, you're going to end up like one of the behemoths in the magazines. With that being said, let's get back to the supplements.

Along with protein supplements, there are many great products that can assist you with achieving your physique dreams. Many products offer promises of huge pecs, bulging biceps, and monstrous quads, so how do we sift through the garbage claims and bogus promises? How do we know what's worth trying? I have narrowed the list down for you as to what may or may not be worth trying to help you achieve your muscle gaining goals.

Protein Types

We all know that protein is the key to muscle gain. After all, protein is made up of amino acids, and so is muscle tissue. The question is what kind of protein we should take. Well, it all depends on how and when you want to use it. There are different types of protein better suited for certain situations than for others. I will not bore you with the science of it all, but it's simple to understand that, in order to gain muscle, you must eat protein.

If I were to ask someone what type of protein they use, more often than not their response will be whey protein. If I were to go one step further and ask what type of whey protein they use, this question is usually answered with a stammer—"Ummm, brand X." Although that wouldn't necessarily be a wrong answer, it's not the answer I was looking for.

Now this is an area where things can become confusing for everyone. There are different types of protein, either slow- or fast-digesting. Within those types, there are different grades of protein, too.

What? You mean that all proteins are not created equal?

Hardly.

Whey Protein Concentrate

Of the three types of whey, concentrate is the *least expensive* to manufacture and, as such, is a highly popular ingredient in the marketing of protein powders. It contains a low level of fat and cholesterol. The thing about concentrates is that they can range anywhere from 29 percent to 89 percent protein by weight. The remainder is lactose, or milk sugar. Chances are that, if you are getting stomach distress from drinking your protein shake, you probably have a cheaper grade of whey protein concentrate. Whey protein concentrate is a fast-digesting protein.

Whey Protein Isolate

Whey isolates are a purer form of whey, generally ranging from 90+ percent protein by weight. They are more expensive to manufacture, thus the higher cost you pay to get a higher isolate content in your protein powder. Whey protein isolate is also a fast-digesting protein.

Whey Protein Hydrolysate

The most costly of the whey proteins to manufacture and the least used of the three, hydrolysate is predigested isolate. This is done through an enzyme process, breaking the isolates down into an even easier form to utilize. Hydrolysates have an extremely bitter taste, and it is difficult to cover up the taste. With the taste and the high manufacturing cost, companies tend not to use this type of whey. Whey protein hydrolysate is also a fast-digesting protein. If you find a protein powder with whey protein hydrolysate as one of the primary ingredients, be prepared to pay significantly more for it.

It should be mentioned that digesting a protein *too quickly* can also lead to stomach and gastrointestinal (GI) distress. While this doesn't necessarily mean you have a cheaper grade of protein, it is still uncomfortable. You should still be aware of the primary protein to determine an overall quality of your supplement.

Casein/Caseinates

Casein is a protein found in milk. It is commonly used as a meal replacement or before bedtime due to its slow digestion rate. This works well because you are not eating for a long time while you sleep. The slow digestion of casein helps you get a constant release of amino acids during that time.

Milk Protein Concentrate

Milk protein concentrate is produced by filtering, evaporating, and drying skim milk. It contains both casein and whey protein. Milk protein concentrate, much like whey protein concentrate, is available in a range of protein levels from 42 percent to 85 percent. The lower the percentage of protein, the higher the percentage of lactose.

Milk Protein Isolate

Much like the forms of whey proteins, milk protein isolate is a more filtered and purified milk protein concentrate. This extra filtration eliminates more of the lactose from the protein, resulting in a higher concentration of protein. Again as with whey, this extra filtration step will cost you more at the store when you make your purchase.

Egg Protein

Eggs have always been an excellent source of protein due to their high biological value (BV) and because they contain all of the essential amino acids. In fact, the BV of eggs is higher than that of any other natural food. This is why eggs have often been considered a "perfect food." They have always been a staple in bodybuilding diets.

Recently, due to avian (bird) flu, the cost to manufacture egg protein powders and the cost of eggs themselves have skyrocketed, causing companies either to discontinue their egg protein powders or significantly raise the price. If you find an egg protein powder at a cheap price, be wary of what you are really buying. Try mixing your egg powder with a little bit of water in a bowl and put it in the microwave. If you have a pure egg powder, it will cook just like a real egg would.

Which Protein Should You Choose?

When you choose which type of protein you want as a supplement, first ask yourself how you are going to use the product. Do you want something for pre- or post-workout? Do you want to use it as a meal replacement? Do you want something before you go to bed? Do you want to just add more protein to your diet?

If you want a protein for pre- or post-workout, you would want to choose a faster-digesting protein to ensure that your muscles are supplied with enough amino acids to help aid recovery and muscle growth from your grueling workouts.

When you want a protein for a meal replacement or before you go to bed, choose one that is slower-digesting to provide a slow, steady supply of amino acids to help pack on new muscle. This slow digestion is similar to eating a whole food meal, which is also beneficial in keeping your insulin levels stable.

When you just want to add more protein to your diet, either of these choices would be fine. Again, ask yourself when you would take the protein to help make a more informed choice.

Some Other Popular Supplements That May Help You Gain Muscle

Creatine

One of the most popular and talked about supplements to come across any gym or muscle magazine, creatine has been a staple supplement for beginners and veterans in their quest for strength and muscle. I will not go into the science of how creatine works, but I will explain the main things to look for when choosing a creatine supplement.

Creatine monohydrate is used very easily by your body. Others may tell you that they have some suped-up version of creatine that blows away monohydrate. We will discuss those, but monohydrate is a tried-and-true form. It just plain works!

You also will want a creatine with little to no sugar. Despite all the ads telling of huge bench presses and gigantic squats due to creatine products loaded with sugar, stay clear of them if you're worried about staying lean while adding muscle. Advertising *hid* these sugars by giving them the name *transporters*. The premise behind this was that the insulin spike caused by the sugars would allow more creatine to be driven into muscle cells. Sugar overloading like that will get you strong, but it'll also get you fat as well. I had to learn that the hard way! I remember when I first tried one of those types of creatine supplements. I did gain a significant amount of strength, but I also gained a significant amount of body fat as well.

If you aren't worried about gaining unsightly fat, these types of products may be for you. Whether it's dextrose, table sugar, or corn syrup, these sugars are too high on the glycemic index and will absolutely lead to excess body fat.

Here's a trick I learned, which you can use when looking at the label of your creatine. When you see a four-pound tub (or whatever the weight may be) of a creatine/sugar mix, look at the total weight (in grams) on the label. Four pounds would be a total weight of 1,816 grams (454 grams/pound).

Now let's say there are sixty servings in the container, with ten grams of creatine per serving. That means that the entire container has only 600 grams of creatine (10 grams x 60 servings = 600 grams). Of that entire 1,816-gram container, 1,216 grams is sugar. That's over *two and a half pounds of sugar!* Now go to the cupboard and find a bag of sugar and ask yourself, "Would I eat this if I wanted to look my absolute best?" When you think of it that way, it changes the way you look at those sugar-loaded products, doesn't it?

Lastly, what you *do* want your creatine to contain is added phosphates. (I know I said I wouldn't get into the science of how creatine works, but this one is important.) When you take in additional creatine, your body needs to have sufficient phosphates for the creatine to bond with in order to produce energy for it to work properly. If there isn't a sufficient amount of phosphates, the additional creatine is excreted, going to waste along with the money you spent on it. However, there is a limit to the amount of creatine your body can store, but that depends on your personal genetics.

I'm often asked if you should "load" creatine. It is not necessary, but you will saturate your muscle cells with the added creatine more quickly when you load than if you do not. Large doses of creatine monohydrate are needed to be effective. (This is the reason most people load when beginning a creatine cycle.) This generally means you will see and feel the results more quickly by loading. It is not necessary, but it is the preferred method most use.

One major point about creatine that needs to be addressed is bloating. If you are getting bloated from using creatine, odds are you don't have pure creatine. It is *impossible* for creatine to make you retain water outside of the muscle unless there are sugars or other additives in your creatine. Pure creatine only holds water in your muscles, which is what you want. All that excess sugar will cause water retention and body fat accumulation.

On that note, don't confuse having body fat with bloating All too often I've heard this mistake. You must realize that pinching body fat is not the same as being bloated. Bloating will go away within hours. Losing body fat will take significantly longer. You must learn to recognize the difference.

Creatine Ethyl Ester

Creatine ethyl ester, or CEE as it is more commonly called, is a new version of creatine made from creatine monohydrate through a chemical process. In the process, an ethyl ester is added to a creatine molecule.

The bonding of particles enhances the absorption rate of creatine and extends its life within your muscle cells. Much like the combination of citrulline and arginine, the combination of ethyl ester and creatine works similarly.

Creatine monohydrate works by drawing water into the muscle cells and enhancing the production of ATP for energy. With CEE, much more creatine will be absorbed because the addition of the ethyl ester allows creatine to pass more easily into the muscle cells.

This all sounds very promising, but unfortunately these claims have not yet been proven.

In one study, two products with CEE were compared to another product only with creatine monohydrate. The results found that CEE is *less stable* than creatine monohydrate, meaning that the CEE compounds were breaking down very rapidly. Also, it was discovered that adding ethyl ester to creatine increased its breakdown to creatinine, a waste byproduct from the energy production process. With this rapid breakdown into creatinine, the body actually has less creatine available.[10]

CEE has yet to be proven as more effective than regular creatine monohydrate. Some companies will advertise how great their new CEE is, but you have to remember that they are trying to make money off of it. Although I have spoken with a few individuals who praised CEE highly, you'll have to judge for yourself.

Creatine Alpha-Ketoglutarate

I'm sure many of you have seen the letters AKG after arginine on most of the nitric oxide products on the market. Now we are starting to see those three letters showing up on the labels of the newest creatine products.

So what does alpha-ketoglutarate or AKG do? Well, when the AKG molecule was first added to arginine, the point was to increase the absorption rate of the amino acid for greater efficiency. The same purpose underlies

---

[10] International Society of Sports Nutrition (2007)

the binding of AKG to creatine. These are the exact same AKG molecules used with both arginine and creatine.

When creatine first burst onto the scene, many people who used it complained of gastrointestinal (GI) upset and diarrhea. (Fortunately, I never had problems with creatine.) Those individuals who had problems did not absorb creatine monohydrate well, and it would sit in their intestines, pulling water into them where it shouldn't be.

To combat this problem, which affected many bodybuilders and fitness enthusiasts alike, alpha-ketoglutarate was added to creatine. AKG is much more easily absorbed by the intestines, which will prevent many GI problems and diarrhea. Furthermore, AKG more easily crosses into muscle tissue *without* the use of creatine transporters, such as simple sugars. Since you are readily absorbing more creatine into your muscle cells, a smaller dosage is just as effective! Your muscles then use the remaining AKG by converting it into creatine phosphate.

AKG is also a precursor to the amino acid glutamine. So in addition to making creatine more effective, you are also getting the added benefits of glutamine. (Glutamine is explained later in this chapter.)

Creatine, combined with AKG, looks to be a great supplement for keeping your energy levels up during your workouts, as well as a quick-energy replenishment between sets. The normal dosage range of creatine AKG is two to five grams per day for the maintenance dose.

Amino Acids

Here is an important fact you should know about amino acids. There is a scientific measure called the Amino Nitrogen/Total Nitrogen rating used to determine the amount of nitrogen in amino acids. The higher the rating, the more effective the amino acid product is. This rating is given by a percentage of the product. The industry average floats at about 12 percent. You will need to ask the manufacturer what its amino nitrogen/total nitrogen rating is.

Here's another trick. When you take your amino acid product, chew one up (if it's a tablet). If it has a sweet or almost pleasant taste, you probably bought something cheap with fillers or sugars, not a quality hydrolysate amino acid. The process to make quality amino acid tablets with a high nitrogen rating will make them taste extremely bitter.

All amino acids are present in muscle tissue, but I will focus only on those most beneficial to building muscle. These are known as the critical cluster, a term explained in chapter 1.

Arginine

Arginine's effectiveness against fat loss has already been explained, but let me tell you how arginine works to make nitric oxide to provide you with *killer pumps* in the gym!

Nitric oxide is formed by a chemical reaction between oxygen and arginine. The production of nitric oxide causes your blood vessels to relax, thus expanding them to allow increased blood flow. More blood flowing through your veins means more blood is going to your muscles while you work out. This means a *better and longer pump*.

More blood going to your muscles also means that you are transporting more nutrients (i.e., amino acids) to your muscle cells, thus making it easier to gain muscle!

The amount of arginine recommended for gaining muscle is the same as it is for fat loss; 2000 mg–3000 mg per day. For better pumps, arginine is usually taken on an empty stomach thirty to forty-five minutes prior to your workouts.

Glutamine

Glutamine is also considered a conditionally essential amino acid. Glutamine aids the immune system and brain function and is the most abundant amino acid in your body. If glutamine is the most abundant amino acid in the body—but under intense stress your body cannot make enough—that means you are burning up glutamine at a very rapid rate! It only makes sense that you should supplement with glutamine! Supplementing with glutamine will aid a healthy immune system, increase mental alertness, and help fight off fatigue. Glutamine will also help stop muscle breakdown brought on from intense training.

The dosage of glutamine varies depending on your specific needs, but anywhere from two to fifteen grams per day would be a good starting point. Generally, it is not needed to be supplemented on non-training days.

I have known some competitors to take a small dosage of glutamine between meals each day while they are dieting for a contest. This practice is usually done throughout the last four weeks of dieting. Individuals on such a diet have claimed that they held on to more muscle for their show. The downside is that any extra glutamine is stored in your liver and can actually slow down your fat-burning process. It's up to your own personal genetics to decide whether this route is best for you.

Branched Chain Amino Acids (BCAA)

There are only three BCAAs: leucine, isoleucine, and valine. These three combined make up one-third of your skeletal muscle. I will use an old analogy here: if your muscle was a brick wall, every third brick would be a branched chain amino acid.

The BCAAs are unlike other amino acids in that they do not have to go through the liver to be metabolized. Instead, they go straight to your muscles. BCAAs are anti-catabolic and have energy-producing effects in the body. Diets high in BCAAs can stimulate insulin production, which in turn increases amino acid uptake. They prevent muscle wasting (very important if you are on a low calorie diet) and have an important role in nitrogen retention.

When your glycogen levels are depleted, supplemental BCAAs can make up a large percentage of your body's energy needs, sparing your hard-earned muscle.

Here's how. When you are on a calorie restricted diet, your body will look for another energy source once your glycogen is used up for your energy needs—*it looks at muscle!* Out of all the amino acids in your muscle, BCAAs are wanted the most as that energy source. Having enough available in your bloodstream will allow your muscle to be spared, and the remaining amino acids will be used to gain new muscle. Leucine is particularly important in this aspect.

The BCAAs also aid in fat loss. Research has shown that subjects on a low-calorie diet high in BCAAs had a higher overall weight loss and body fat reduction, as well as *greater fat loss from the abdominal area.*[11]

As if all of these benefits of BCAA supplementation weren't enough, they also have been shown to be a "brain-booster." The BCAAs prevent the amino acid tryptophan from entering the brain, where it is then converted to serotonin. Serotonin makes you feel happy and content, but also tired and sleepy. Remember after your big Thanksgiving dinner, how tired you felt? That's because turkey is high in tryptophan! Plus, all the extra carbs you probably ate had allowed tryptophan easier entry into your brain. (But that's another story and outside the scope of this book.)

When you choose a BCAA product, you always want to make sure that the dosage of leucine is twice that of the other two BCAAs. Leucine helps start protein synthesis at an earlier stage than the other amino acids. Research has shown that taking leucine alone is not adequate to get results. The typical dose for the BCAAs is five to twenty grams per day depending on your body weight.

I can honestly tell you that BCAAs are my personal favorite supplement. Whether trying to gain muscle, lose fat, or just perk up for a while, they truly are an amazing supplement.

Gamma Oryzanol
Recently, gamma oryzanol exploded with wild popularity onto the supplement scene, with its claims of increased

---

[11]   American Journal of Physiology, Endocrinology and Metabolism (2003)

testosterone levels, muscle mass, and energy. But is all this hype really reliable? Let's take a closer look at this supplemental wonder.

Gamma oryzanol is a mixture of *ferulic acid* esters (i.e., chemical compounds) derived from rice bran oil and other grain oils. In plants, it serves as an antioxidant within cells. In Japan, it has been used as a medicine; it was first used to treat anxiety. During the 1970s, gamma oryzanol was found to be an effective treatment in women suffering from symptoms of menopause. It also has been used to combat high cholesterol and triglyceride levels.

In the bodybuilding and fitness world, gamma oryzanol has become extremely popular because it is believed to have *steroid-mimicking* properties. Such properties include an increase in growth hormone output, as well as higher testosterone production. More testosterone means more muscle!

Unfortunately, these claims in human studies are yet to be proven. Some studies have shown that gamma oryzanol has a poor absorption rate, with most of the supplement excreted as waste.

It would seem, however, that higher doses of gamma oryzanol have no effect while a smaller dose does seem more beneficial. In a study with bodybuilders taking 30 mg per day over an eight-week period, all subjects showed an increase in body weight and strength. Another study used 500 mg per day over nine weeks. Subjects taking gamma oryzanol showed no difference in weight or strength compared to those who just took a placebo.[12]

---

[12] International Journal of Sports Nutrition (1997)

In studies conducted on animals, gamma oryzanol has actually been shown to suppress leutinizing hormone, (a hormone involved in testosterone production), reduce growth hormone levels and reduce testosterone production!

Though many swear by it, there is no conclusive evidence showing that gamma oryzanol lives up to its hype as an effective muscle-building supplement. Again, you will have to judge this one for yourself.

Since it is made up of ferulic acid, you may want to try supplementing with that instead. In animal studies, ferulic acid was shown to be effective at converting more of the food ingested into body weight.[13] Ferulic acid may also be a less expensive substitute for gamma oryzanol although there is no conclusive evidence for that claim, either.

A daily dose of ferulic acid would be about 10 mg–60 mg.

Colostrum
Often acclaimed as an incredible muscle builder, colostrum is, in essence, *strong milk*. It is produced during pregnancy in both humans and bovine animals.

The human form of colostrum, which is given to infants during breast-feeding in the mother's milk, is high in concentrations of carbohydrates, protein, and antibodies. It is also low in fat.

The bovine form of colostrum, which is the type used in supplements, is a very rich source of growth factors. This has made it ideal for use in muscle-gaining

---

[13] International Journal of Sports Nutrition (1997)

supplements, as well as on its own. The most prominent of these growth factors is Insulin-like Growth Factor 1, which we'll refer to as IGF-1. IGF-1 is a hormone which has *highly anabolic effects*. It has the ability to stimulate protein synthesis, as well as inhibit protein breakdown. This means that your body absorbs more protein into its muscles while less muscle tissue is broken down. A big advantage to anyone looking to gain more muscle! Bovine colostrum contains one of the highest concentrations of IGF-1 in nature, and studies do show that bovine colostrum supplementation in athletes does increase the levels of IGF-1 concentrations in the bloodstream. This increase helps improve endurance and performance and has other positive effects on health.

In one study on colostrum, subjects were told to do aerobic exercise and weight training at least three times per week over the course of eight weeks. Those supplementing with colostrum showed a *significant increase* in lean body mass!

Although the research on colostrum is limited,[14] it does show signs of serious promise. There are no reported negative side effects of colostrum supplementation.

The dosage range of liquid colostrum in these studies was 25 ml to 125 ml per day or twenty to sixty grams per day in a powder form.

Tribulus Terrestris
Tribulus terrestris stakes its claim as both a booster of sex drive and an agent to help raise testosterone levels. It is

---

[14] University of Delaware – Sports Science Laboratory (2001); Mero et al. (1997)

also thought that it can aid in the increase of lean body mass.

While tribulus terrestris has been used since the 1970s to aid an individual's sex drive, its ability to raise testosterone levels is doubtful. Studies have shown that, while it may raise testosterone levels, it still leaves them within the *normal* range. It may be useful to those with below normal testosterone levels. (You can consult your doctor to have a blood test taken to determine your testosterone levels.)

In a four-week study of tribulus terrestris, subjects were given 10 mg–20 mg daily per kilogram of body weight. The results concluded that it had no effect on male sex hormones.

Fifteen subjects in another study were either given 3.21 mg of tribulus per kilogram of body weight or a placebo. They were tested over eight weeks using resistance training. After that time, neither body weight nor the body fat percentage of subjects in either group changed.[15]

Another study included twenty-two male athletes given either 450 mg of tribulus each day or a placebo over a five-week period of heavy strength training. After the study had ended, both groups experienced a significant increase in strength and lean body mass. However, there was no difference between the two groups, meaning that, while both groups got stronger and more muscular, neither group outperformed the other as far as results. [16]

---

[15] International Journal of Sports Nutrition and Exercise Metabolism (2000)

[16] Southern Cross University Lismore, New South Wales, Australia (2007)

I have used a popular tribulus terrestris supplement in the past. I can tell you that I didn't notice anything significant from the product. Needless to say, it was a one-time deal for me, and I've since then never used another tribulus terrestris supplement.

There have been reports of a toxic effect in sheep although no serious side effects have been shown in human studies. Some more mild effects of tribulus terrestris supplementation have been the following: more energy (though I would consider that a good side effect), feeling warmer, a slightly faster heart rate, and some restlessness.

Usual dosage ranges of tribulus terrestris are around 250 mg taken three times per day. The above side effects have been more prominent at dosages of 500 mg per day and higher..

Some Final Thoughts

So there you have it. Some of the most well-kept and unknown tricks of the trade in the supplement industry, as well as additional information on some of the more highly marketed supplements.

I hope that you have found this book's information eye-opening and insightful. It was a great joy to be able to help you gain some new knowledge so that you can make better-informed decisions when purchasing your supplements.

This is not the be-all and end-all to supplement guides, but the points made here are those which, I believe, every purchaser of supplements should be made aware. Whether you are an avid competitor or you are just starting your journey to change your physique, I hope you have learned something helpful. The supplement world is constantly changing and making new progress and new products. Do your research to find out what really shows potential and what is mostly hype. Don't jump the gun in order to be in on the latest fad of supplement popularity.

There are a lot of dirty tricks played on the unaware consumer, but I hope that that is no longer the case for you. You should now be ready with your newfound knowledge to go out and effectively choose which supplements you should spend your money on to get the results you have been striving for.

I wish you the best in health!